Disease and Parasite Prevention in Farm Animals: Ten Major Steps

by

D.E. Goodman, DVM

Christian Veterinary Mission

Christian Veterinary Mission

Current Book Information at:
www.cvm.org

Library of Congress Cataloging-in-Publication Data

Goodman, D. E.
Disease and parasite prevention in farm animals : ten major steps / D.E. Goodman.
p. cm. -- (Special topics series ; mini-bk. no. 1)
ISBN 1-886532-17-6
1. Veterinary medicine. 2. Livestock--Diseases--Prevention.
3. Veterinary parasitology. I. Title. II. Series: Special topics series (Seattle, Wash.) ; mini-bk. no. 1.
SF745.G59 2006
636.089'4--dc22

2006013916

This is the first book in a series of Mini-Books that we hope will deal with special problems of livestock production. The issues dealt with in the Disease and Parasite book are costly to many farmers throughout the world. We believe the suggestions for dealing with the problems are practical and effective. If you have other issues you would like for us to develop a book on, please be sure and send your suggestions to CVM.

Raising Healthy Animals Series

Every year, thousands of people around the world struggle to survive because they don't have the right knowledge, skills and resources to care for their animals. Christian Veterinary Mission (CVM) sends veterinary professionals to live and work alongside many of these people to encourage them and provide them with not only much needed veterinary expertise, but also the hope that is only found in Christ. CVM veterinarians build lasting relationships with individuals and communities, helping them be transformed through Christ's love.

CVM, in its effort to be meaningfully involved in work in the developing world, quickly found there was little appropriate educational material available. CVM set about developing basic resource materials in animal husbandry for farmers and agricultural workers. Apparently, they met a real need, as these books have been accepted throughout the developing nations of the world.

The series of books published by Christian Veterinary Mission includes the following in order of publication:

Raising Healthy Pigs *	Drugs and Their Usage
Raising Healthy Rabbits *	Where There Is No Animal Doctor
Raising Healthy Fish	Raising Healthy Horses
Raising Healthy Cattle	Zoonoses: Animal Diseases That Affect Humans
Raising Healthy Poultry *+	Raising Healthy Honey Bees
Raising Healthy Goats *	Slaughter and Preservation of Meat
Raising Healthy Sheep	Disease and Parasite Prevention in Farm Animals

[Also available in: * Spanish + French].

CVM fieldworkers have also developed specific training materials for the countries in which they work.

All of these books have been put together by Christian men and women; in a labor of love and service, for people in need throughout the world. It demonstrates dedication to their profession, service to humanity and a witness to their faith. We hope that they are a help to you in developing an appropriate livestock program to meet your needs. We pray God's blessing on their use.

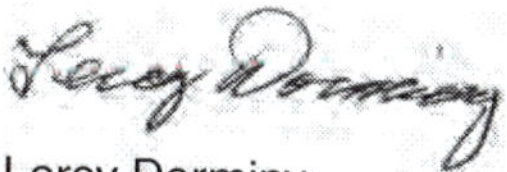

Leroy Dorminy
CVM Founder

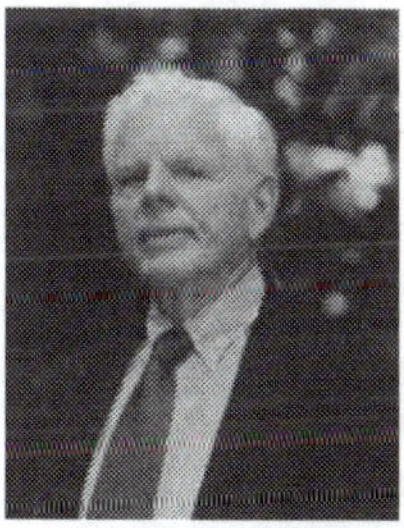

Table of Contents

Section I
Background and Introduction....................................5

1.1 About the Book....................................5
1.2 How to Use This Book....................................6
1.3 About the Author....................................7
1.4 About the Illustrator....................................8

Section II
10 Steps to Parasite and Disease Prevention on Small Farms....................................9

1. Locating Livestock and Poultry Facilities....................................10
2. Managing Pens and Pastures for Swine, Poultry, and Horses....................................12
3. Managing Pastures for Ruminants....................................15
4. Using Temporary and Movable Buildings....................................18
5. Using the Cleanest Areas for Birthing....................................20
6. Providing Clean Drinking Water....................................22
7. Using Proper Feeding Techniques....................................25
8. Protecting Animals from Environmental Extremes....................................27
9. Separating Healthy and Sick Animals....................................29
10. Properly Disposing of Dead Animals....................................31

Section III
Special Notes on Poultry Disease and Parasite Prevention....................................32

Section IV
Discussion on Raising Animals Off Ground....................................34

1. Drawbacks to Raising Animals Off Ground....................................34
2. Situations in Which Raising Animals Off Ground is Beneficial....................................35

Summary....................................36

Section I

Background and Introduction

1.1 About the Book

"Why do our farm animals get sick and how can we keep them healthy?"

This is a question veterinarians and other specialists who work with small farmers hear frequently. Most of these farmers work very hard, giving time, effort, and loving care to their animals in the hope that their farm will be more productive.

Yet, very often, their animals and poultry are much less healthy and productive than they could be. Too often, we see death, chronic stunting, sickly newborns, and many other signs of poor health. So, why is this? What can farmers and those who advise them do about these problems?

In this small book are suggestions for raising healthier animals on small farms. While not all of these methods will apply in every area or situation, much of the information can be of help on most farms. If these principles are applied, livestock health and farm efficiency will improve.

Amazingly, most of these practices cost very little and are simple enough for farmers to carry out themselves or with the help of farm workers or family.

It is very important to remember that the information and methods discussed in this book cannot replace parasite treatment and vaccination. But, if these methods are used together with vaccination, animals will be healthier.

Unfortunately, modern vaccines and treatments are often unavailable or unaffordable for small farmers. And, if proper preventive procedures are not used, vaccinated animals may become ill anyway.

The background, methods, concepts, and practices in this book are based on the author's lifetime of personal interest and experience. While this information would be particularly applicable to poultry and other birds, it can be useful in raising all farm animal species.

1.2 How to Use This Book

This book was written for those who train farmers in developing countries. The author hopes that those who read and learn from this book will teach others.

This book could also be valuable to small farmers as a primer (beginning book) in developing areas without trained agricultural workers or veterinarians. The material in this book may be effectively taught using the methods suggested in "Learning Together: The Agricultural Worker's Participatory Sourcebook," available from CVM.

Christian Veterinary Mission and the author hope that the material in this book is informative and presented in a simple and readable form.

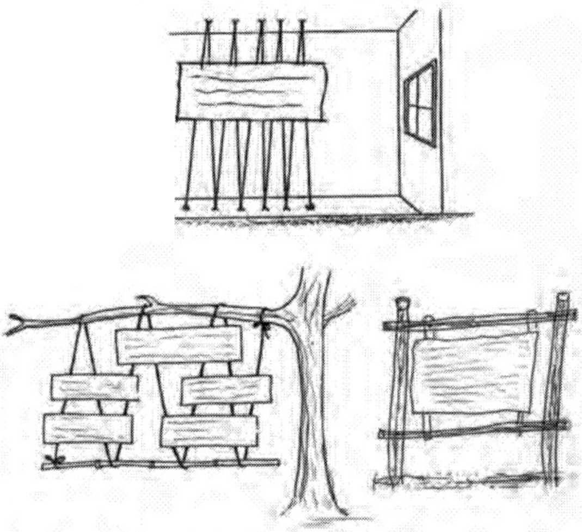

These types of displays would be useful for a trainer teaching in a developing country. They can be easily made with sticks and rope.

1.3 About the Author

Dr. D.E. Goodman has traveled widely, living, working, and teaching in developing areas of the world. In addition to his extensive personal experience in animal production on small farms, he has been involved in rural veterinary practice and served as an animal health consultant. For many years, he worked in animal disease prevention, control, and eradication for Clemson University.

Dr. Goodman is also the author of "Raising Healthy Pigs on Small Farms", the first in a very successful series of animal health books published by Christian Veterinary Mission (CVM). Currently, he serves as the content editor of "International Animal Health News", a quarterly publication of CVM.

He and his family live in rural South Carolina where they participate in church and community affairs and farming.

1.4 About the Illustrator

The majority of the illustrations in this booklet were provided by Dr. Beth Robinson. Beth has recently returned to veterinary relief work in the Dallas/Ft. Worth area, mainly with dogs and cats. She began raising goats several years ago as a 4-H project for her children and finds she really enjoys working with them (the goats and the children).

She and her husband Don look forward to his retirement when they will be able to participate in mission trips and Habitat for Humanity building projects.

1.5 About the Editors

Two key individuals worked as editors of this booklet.

- Dr. Kelly Ward lives in Idaho and has edited several books for CVM. She is also involved with veterinary students at Washington State University, and she is actively involved with her family in church and community activities.

- Miss Rose Hurley graduated from University of Washington and is now studying linguistics at a graduate level in Israel. Rose was active in 4-H while growing up, and she has special interests in animal health activities.

Section II

10 Steps to Parasite and Disease Prevention

With all the advances in technology over the years, we often lose sight of those basic principles and practices that can help small farmers raise healthy animals.

Too often, new medicines and products are not available to small farmers. Or, if they are, they are too expensive to be widely used. In such cases, we can turn to simple and inexpensive preventive methods.

These practices alone will not prevent all diseases and health problems. But, they can greatly increase the benefits of vaccination and medication. And, in situations where modern vaccines are not readily available, following these methods will help the small farmer to raise healthy animals.

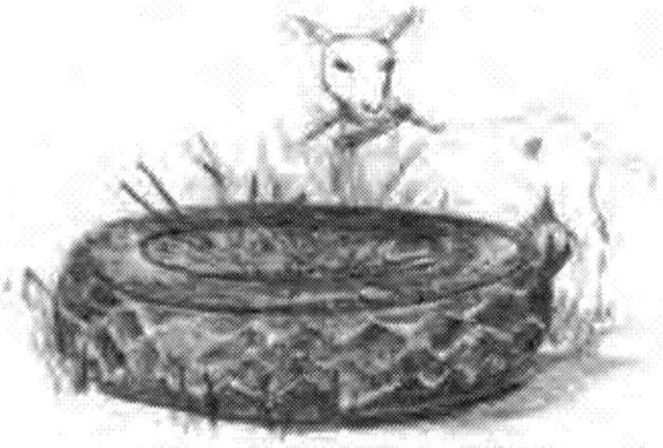

Parasites and disease causing germs are common in food kept near the ground. This goat may become ill from his feed.

Step 1. Locating Livestock and Poultry Facilities

The location of the livestock unit, regardless of its size, is of extreme importance.

In low, wet land or areas where there is standing water, disease germs and parasite eggs survive much longer than they could on high, dry land exposed to sunlight. And, because animals often drink from such areas, livestock often become infected. Also, animals often defecate and urinate where they drink. This allows disease germs and ova (eggs) to be passed from a sick animal to a healthy animal that drinks the affected water or eats food containing these germs. For example, a parasite like hookworm is spread when ova (eggs) hatch and become free swimming larvae (small, immature worms). This parasite has the ability to penetrate the skin of an animal as it drinks or grazes. Other parasites, like biting insects that suck blood and spread disease, also live in low, wet areas. Additionally, feed kept in moist places is very likely to contain dangerous germs and parasite eggs.

To prevent such problems, it is generally better to use high, drier areas for animals. In some situations, however, these areas may have less protection from wind and sun. If so, we may have to provide temporary protection from extreme weather until trees can be grown, providing more permanent cover. Another consideration in moving animals to the drier land is water that was previously supplied by surface water must be provided for animals. In spite of these challenges, it is often worthwhile to keep animals on the higher, drier areas of a farm whenever possible.

On some farms, there will be very limited dry land for animal production. In these cases, it is necessary to adequately drain lower, wet lands by digging trenches (small shallow ditches) through pens and pastures and then surrounding them with larger ditches. In general, areas where surface water remains for more than a few days at a time are not safe for raising animals.

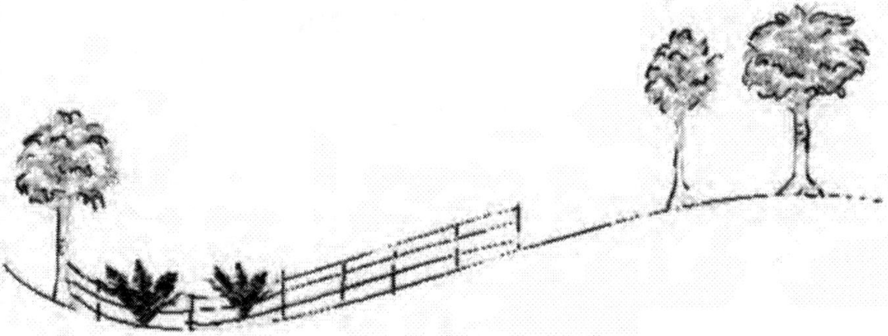

This farm is NOT recommended.

- The pen is in a low, wet area
- Animals will drink the standing water and their feed will be moist.

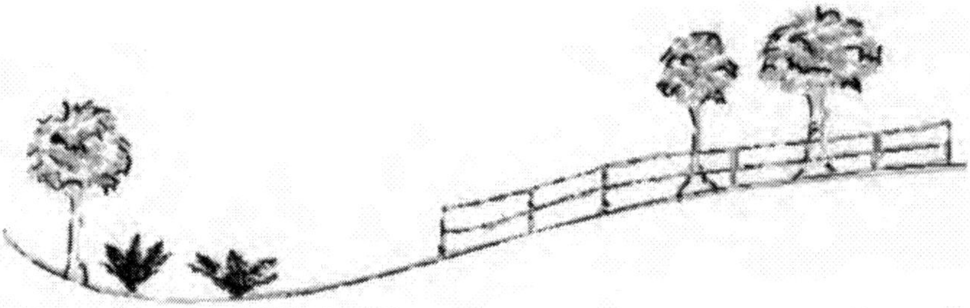

This farm uses the land well

- The animal will live in a high, dry area
- There is adequate shade and no standing water, feed will stay dry

Step 2. Managing Pens and Pastures for Swine, Poultry, and Horses

One of the most important and necessary methods for preventing parasites and disease is that of pen and pasture rotation. This is a long standing and well proven method that should be used by farmers everywhere in the world.

Small farmers and those who advise them must always remember that feces and filth often contain dangerous germs and worm (internal parasite) eggs or larvae. These creatures can live and continue to cause health problems for a long time. Often, a pen has been used continually for many years and is so dirty and contaminated that it is almost impossible to raise healthy animals in it. In addition, using a pasture for long periods can be harmful. For instance, horses that graze too long in one place are more likely to take in sand and develop digestive problems. Likewise, excessive grazing often results in poor recovery of the land.

To prevent such problems, one should periodically move animals and poultry from areas that have been in use for a long time. When animals are moved to an area not previously used, they will not be exposed to filth and feces with disease causing germs and eggs. Transferring livestock to a cleaner area, even if it is only a short distance away, often results in great improvement in the health of the animals, especially of the young.

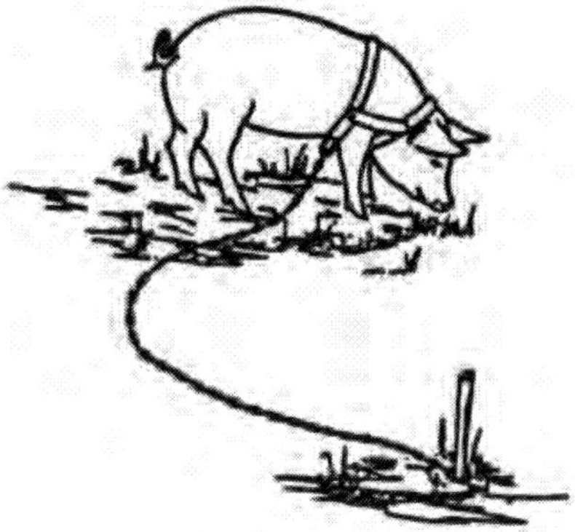

Tethering is another way to rotate grazing areas. It is a good system for the farmer who is not able to fence his land.

Usually, a "double" or "use one, rest one" pen or pasture rotation is the most practical system. In this arrangement, one pasture area or pen is left unused while the other houses the livestock. This allows time for many of the disease germs and parasite eggs in the soil to die before they can infect livestock.

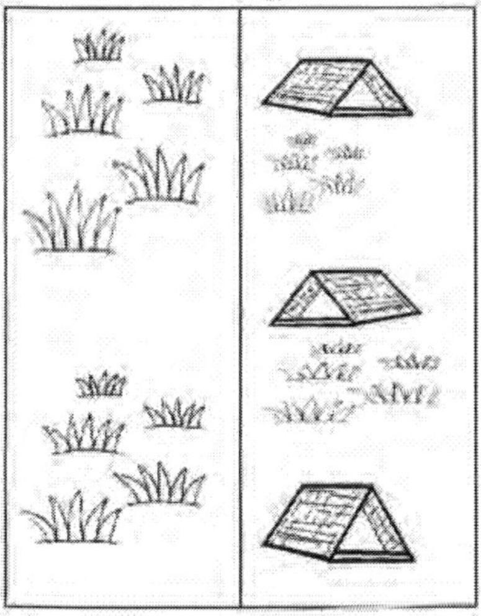

This drawing illustrates the "double" or "use one, rest one" system of rotation. The land is divided into separate pastures. There are temporary buildings in the active pasture, while the resting pasture is left empty. After a few weeks, the buildings and animals should be moved to the rested land.

In some extreme situations, when pastures have been heavily used for long periods of time, it may be necessary to use a "triple" or "use one, rest two" system. In this system, pasture land is divided into three sections, and only one is used at a time, while the other two sections rest. This allows each section of pasture to rest twice as long, and reduces the number of germs and parasite eggs. This is the best method for on farms that have experienced many health problems. If the pastures are low or wet, the "triple" method is also recommended.

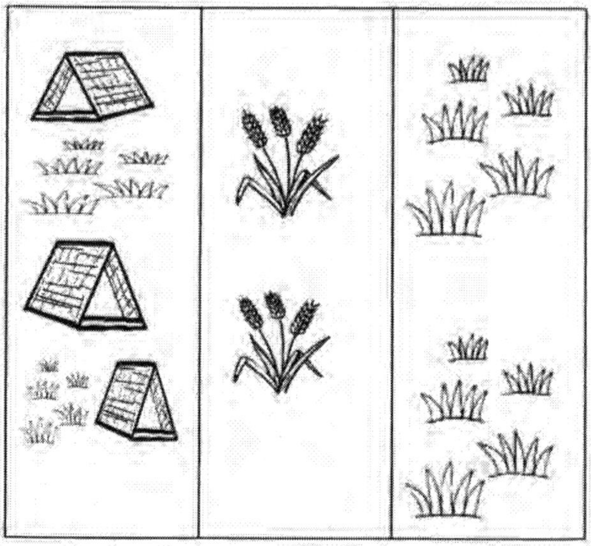

In the "Use One, Rest Two" or "Triple" System, pictured above, each pasture is rested for a longer period of time after being used for animals.

Step 3. Managing Pastures for Ruminants

Without frequent pasture rotation, animals like cattle, sheep, llamas, and goats may "over-graze" an area. How do you know that animals are "overgrazing"? If they are, there will be bare spots of soil in the field. Overgrazing is a serious problem because it harms the land. If an area is overgrazed, it will not recover quickly and you may not be able to use it for a long time. In addition, animals eating on bare, overgrazed ground often ingest dangerous parasite eggs.

So, there are two reasons to alternate ruminants' pastures. First, it gives the land time to recover and for the pasture to grow back. Secondly, it disrupts the life cycle of many common parasites. When land is left empty, particularly with exposure to sunlight, the immature parasites in the soil dry out and die.

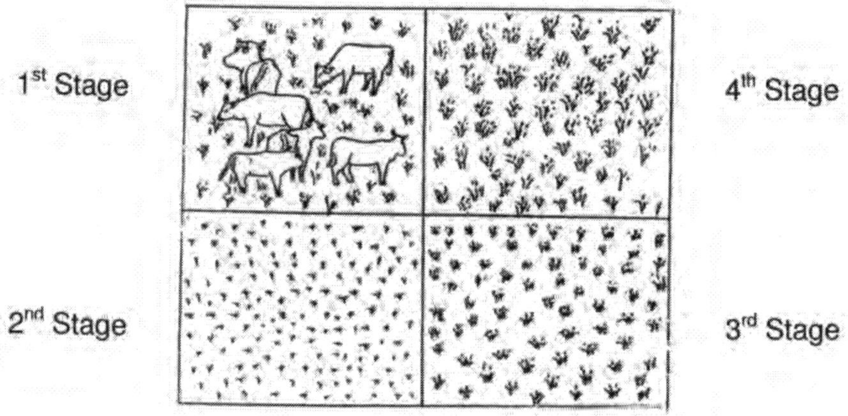

This is an excellent plan for pasture rotation. Pastures are allowed to rest for long periods between use. The resting areas may be used to grow crops.

Many factors must be considered when deciding how often to rotate pastures. The number of pastures available, the number of animals grazing, and the fertility of the land will all affect how often a piece of land can be used. In general, it is good to rest an area for about three weeks. But, each farmer should find the method that works best for his land and animals.

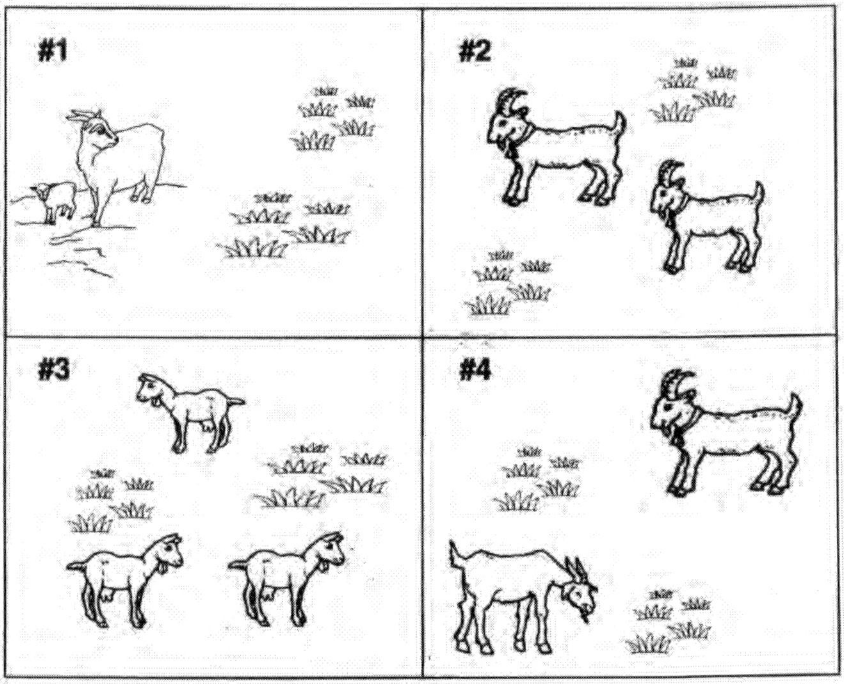

1. **Keep babies and mothers separate from other animals and on the cleanest, least used land.**
2. **Keep separate pens for breeding males**
3. **Keep pregnant animals on pastures with enough space to give birth.**
4. **Keep young, weaned animals separate**

These drawings show different ways to manage land on a farm. Land can be divided into separate pens and pastures. Animals can be moved from used pastures to fresh, rested ones. Temporary buildings would be placed in the new pens and pastures. Notice how animals are kept in small, separate groups to stop disease from spreading and to protect young animals from parasites. Again, this picture does not need to be followed exactly; it is just an example of good pasture rotation.

If possible, reserve a little extra pasture area so that it will be available in dry periods. Hay can be made from this land and stored for emergency feed.

Fertilization is another method for improving ruminants' pastures. In many areas commercial fertilizers are not available and animal manure or compost works well. In other areas commercial fertilizer is available and can be used effectively if proper soil testing is available. There may be government or university personnel who are able to assist the small farmer with this testing. Although fertilizer can be expensive or difficult to find, it may increase the yield of a pasture. Also, forage grown with fertilizer is more nutritious than forage grown without fertilizer. Usually, the increase in pasture production and animal health will make up for the cost of the fertilizer.

Step 4. Using Temporary and Movable Buildings

When a farmer uses a building or pasture over a long period of time, his animals will be more likely to develop disease and parasites. The buildup of feces, urine, rotten bedding, waste feed, and moist soil creates a perfect environment for germs and parasites to cause health problems in livestock and poultry. This is especially dangerous for newborn and young animals that have little resistance to these harmful germs.

A simple solution to this problem is to build inexpensive temporary or movable buildings. The use of structures that can either moved and rested or simply be torn down will greatly reduce disease spread.

If it is impossible to use temporary or movable structures, feces and contaminated soil should be removed as often as possible and replaced with clean soil. Ideally, farm animal and poultry buildings should be refreshed twice a year, but even one time a year can improve health. If there is an outbreak of illness or disease, it is essential that the affected building be cleaned and disinfected soon afterward.

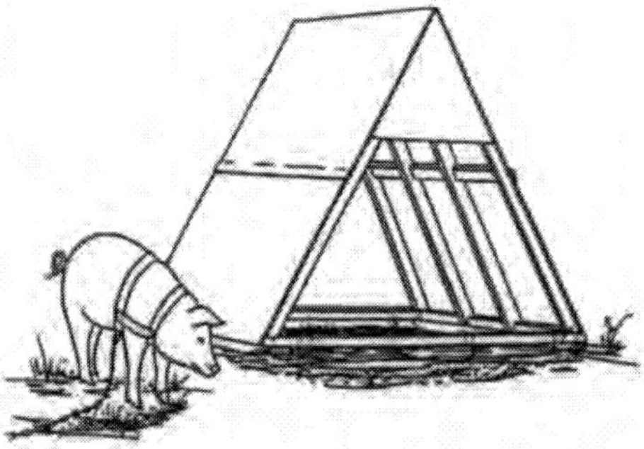

This shed was built on pieces of wood so that it can be easily moved.
In summer, the ends are left open so air can flow through.
In winter, one or both ends can be covered to protect the animals from cold winds.

During the cleaning process, after the dirty soil has been removed, the building should be thoroughly wetted down with soap, water, and disinfectant if possible.

A simple and inexpensive disinfectant can be made using ¾ cup household chlorine bleach (5.25% sodium hypochlorite active ingredient) per one gallon of water. After cleansing, the doors and windows should be opened to allow sunlight and fresh air into the building. The farmer should wait at least one day after using the disinfectant before bringing in new soil. The building must be completely dry before the animals can safely return.

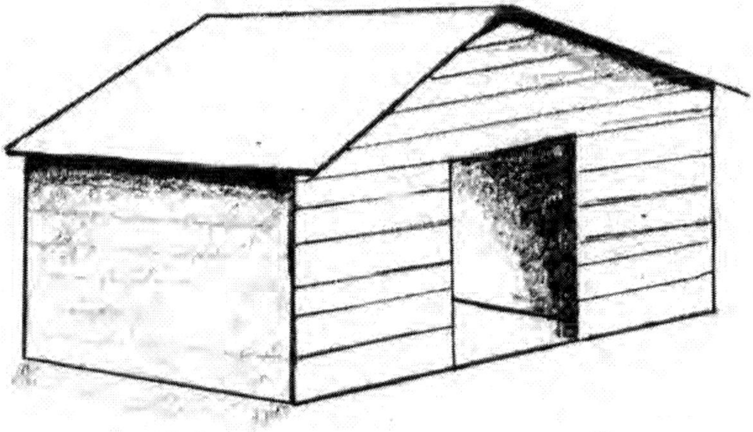

A permanent building like this must be cleaned regularly. It will also be hot in the summer and is too heavy to move.

Always consider using the fecal material removed from the building as fertilizer for crops. Manure should be plowed into the soil several months before the crops are planted for best results. Fecal matter should NOT be applied over crops intended for human consumption.

Step 5. Using the Cleanest Areas for Birthing

Providing a clean area for birthing is a very important way to improve the health of livestock. Fortunately, it is simple to understand and inexpensive to put into use.

On many farms, the same pen, pasture, shed, or stable has been used for many years for birthing and raising young animals. But, the newborn comes into the world with almost no resistance to disease or parasites. From its first breath, it is exposed to a very unhealthy environment filled with feces and filth containing germs and worm eggs. In such a situation, it is almost impossible for the newborn to get a healthy start in life.

So, minimizing the exposure of the newborn and very young animal to illness and parasites is very important. It can mean the difference between a healthy, fast growing creature and a sick, stunted, or dead animal.

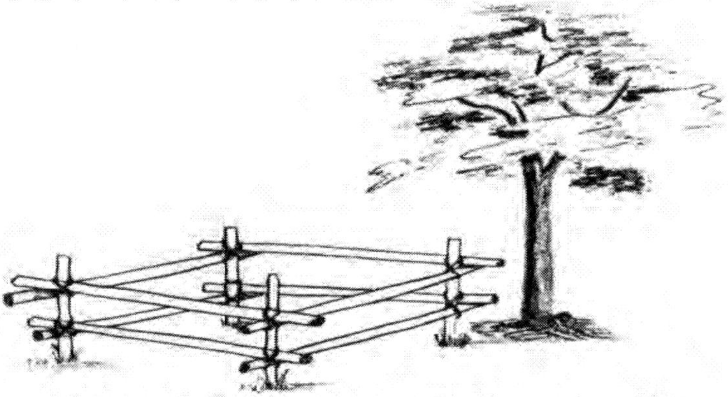

This pen is made of poles joined together with wire or string. It is a simple way to create a clean, safe space for birthing.

In order to protect the newborn, the farmer should use higher, dry land for birthing, whenever possible. Ideally, this should be the area that has been out of use for the longest time so that it will be the least contaminated. If acreage is very limited, the farmer should reserve small pieces of high, drier land exclusively for birthing and raising the newborn. This area should not be used for more than six months at a time. Instead, it should be periodically rested and the birthing area should be moved to another dry, clean piece of land. If there are signs of illness in the newborn or mother, the next birth should take place in another area, and the contaminated pen should not be used for at least a year.

In order to limit exposure to illness and parasites, the birthing area should not be used by older animals.

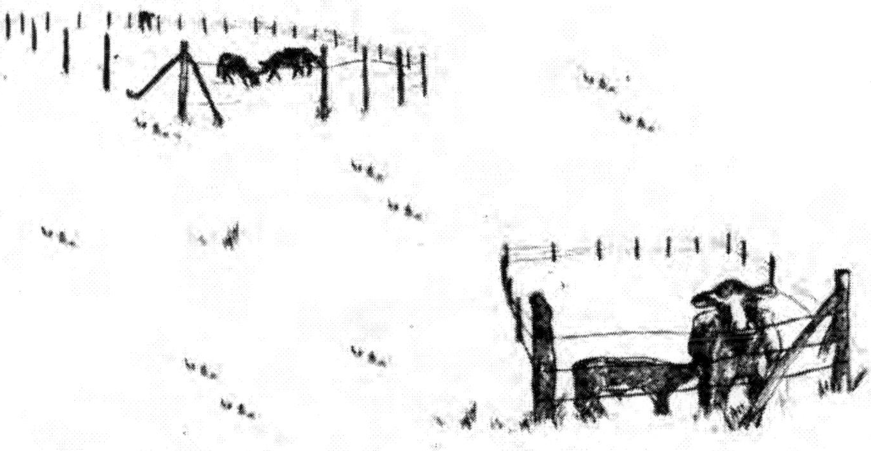

This mother and newborn are kept a safe distance from the rest of the herd.
Move animals to a separate pasture late in their pregnancy so the baby will be born in a clean environment .

In short, since birthing in a clean area is one of the most important things we can do to raise healthy animals, it should be practiced by every animal owner. Those who advise farmers should understand the procedure and speak about it to everyone who raises animals.

Step 6. Providing Clean Drinking Water

Like the other practices outlined in this section, providing fresh, clean drinking water is a simple but important method for improving animal health. In fact, it is one of the most essential factors in raising healthy livestock.

Animals, and in particular pigs, will drink whatever water is available to them. However, they actually prefer clean, fresh water and are much healthier if they have access to it. The nursing female, for example, must have an adequate water supply if she is to provide milk for her newborn. The young animal, too, needs fresh water as it begins to eat solid food.

Although relying on surface water is usually the most convenient option for the small farmer, it has many drawbacks. For instance, the risk of taking in dangerous germs and parasites by mouth is very high when animals are allowed to drink from ponds, surface water, or small streams. Clearly, these water sources should be avoided if at all possible. Likewise, this water often tastes bad to the animal, limiting how much it drinks and negatively affecting health and growth. Dependence on surface water alone can also mean the need for an additional water source due to seasonal problems with availability.

Instead, provide fresh water in a clean trough or container. The location of the drinking trough is essential. In general, water placed close to the food source increases the amount animals eat. If their water it located too far away, they may drink less and lose weight. Placing the water source in a cool, shady area easily accessible to the livestock should result in better growth and overall health.

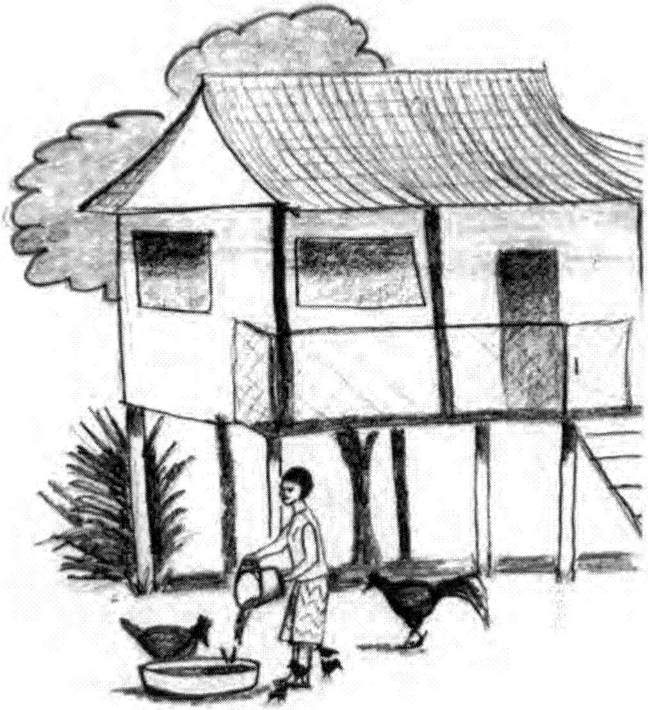

Also, the height of the trough will vary according to the height of the livestock. Cattle and horses will need taller troughs than those designed for pigs. Remember that animals begin to drink water at a very young age and it is important to provide a drinking source that is low enough to the ground for small animals to reach easily.

Waterers

Fig. 5. Chick waterer

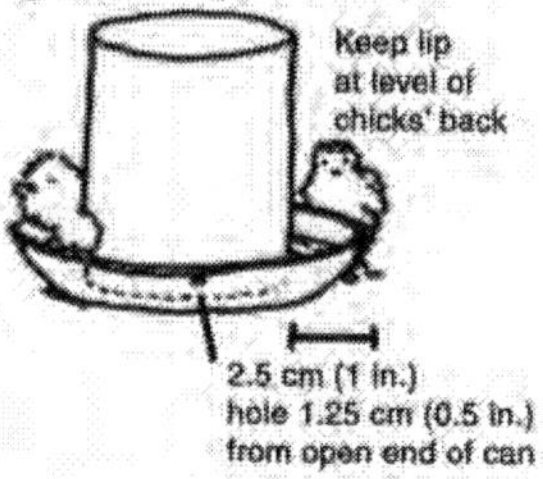

Fig. 6. Parts of a waterer

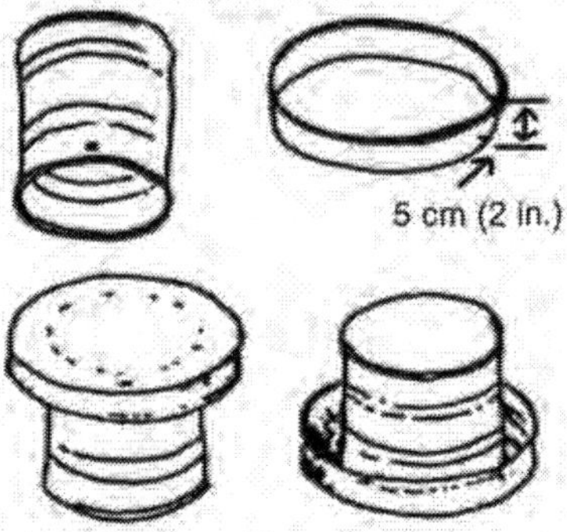

Fig. 7. Clay waterer

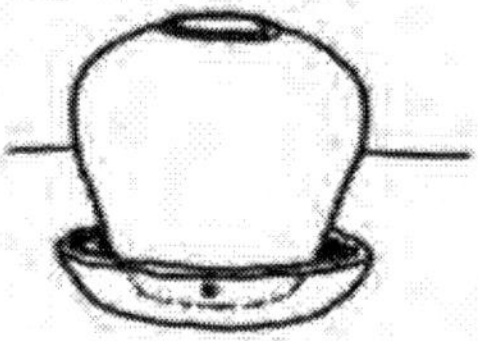

Fig. 8. Bottle waterer

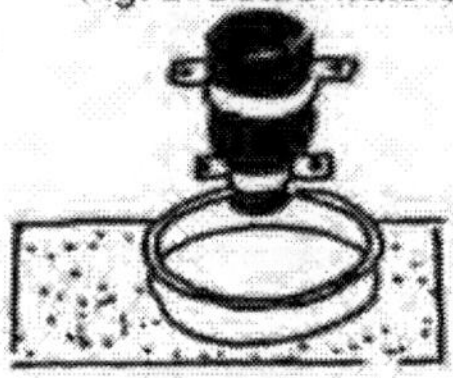

Fig. 9. Gourd waterer

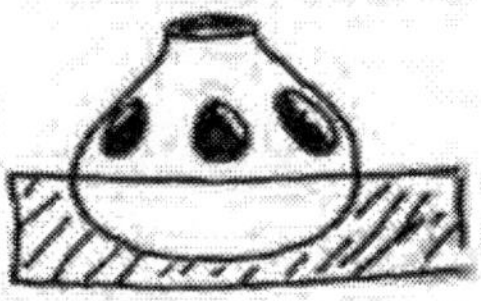

These waterers are designed for chicks and chickens

Outdoor Feeders and Waterers

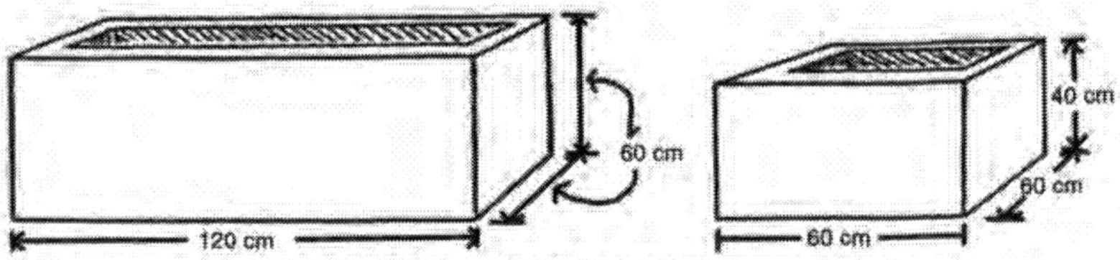

CREEP FEEDER / PIGLET WATERER

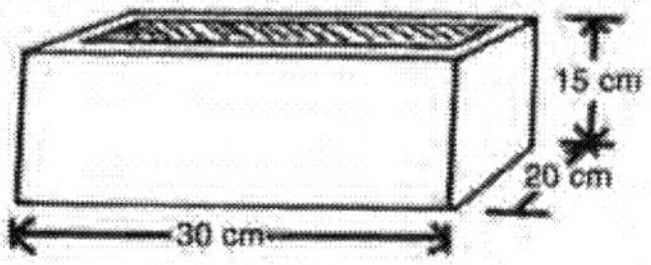

The troughs above have been adjusted for animals of different sizes

Step 7. Using Proper Feeding Techniques

Food that is placed on the ground for eating will most likely contain feces and therefore have a high risk of passing on germs and parasite eggs to the livestock eating it. Likewise, food placed on the ground may spoil more quickly, making the animal sick. This spoiled food will also have lost much of its nutrient content. In addition, there is also significant feed waste from feeding on the ground. This is true for all farm animals, including poultry.

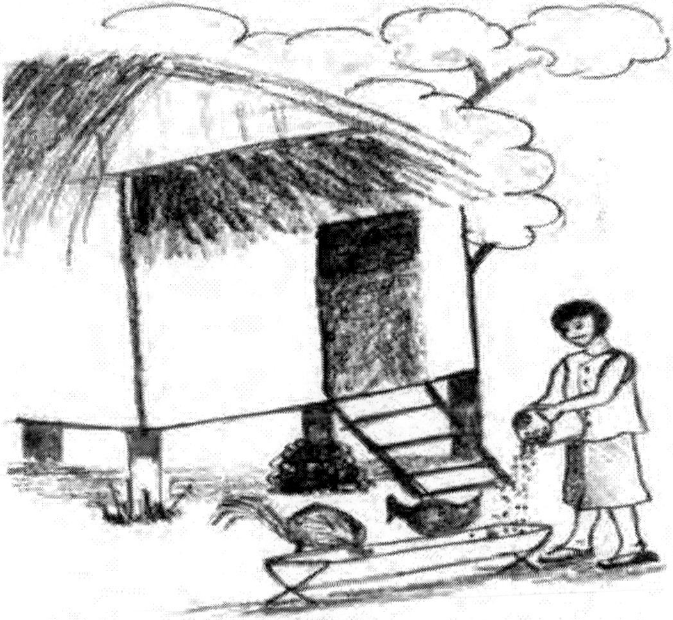

Because they are fed from a trough, these chickens are protected from many diseases

However, with a little thought and the use of inexpensive materials, the small farmers can prevent these problems. Troughs, racks, and other feeding equipment can be made from waste or cheap materials. Tires, inexpensive lumber and metal are commonly used. In some areas, dugout logs are popular for troughs.

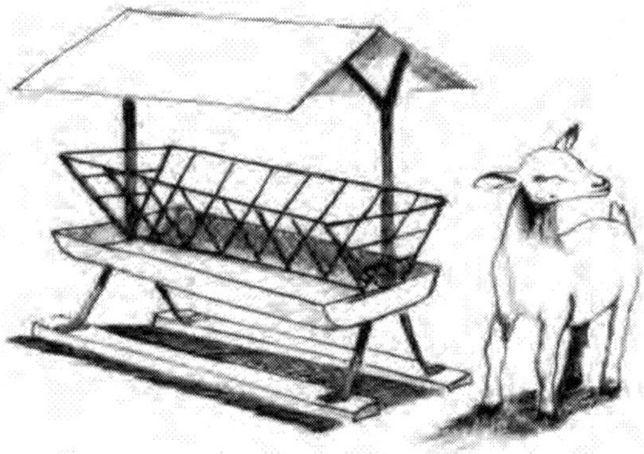

This trough keeps food clean and protected from rain.

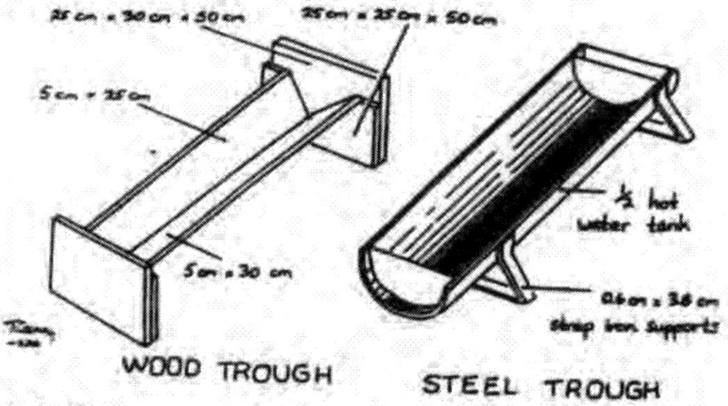

II E-5

These troughs were designed to provide clean water and food for pigs. If they were made wider and higher off the ground, they could also be used for cattle and horses.

It is also possible to tie bundles of grass, leaves and hay and let the bundles hang down from a tree branch or the roof. This keeps the feed from getting dirty on the ground.

The same issues of placement and height discussed for water troughs apply to feeding racks. As a general rule, the feeding equipment should be placed in an easily accessible area and designed to meet the needs of the specific animal on each farm.

Step 8. Protecting Animals from Environmental Extremes

Protecting livestock from extreme weather is another important consideration. Exposure to severe conditions, both hot and cold, can make an animal more susceptible to disease and parasites. So, although many animals can adapt to a wide variety of climates, they still need protection from extreme weather conditions.

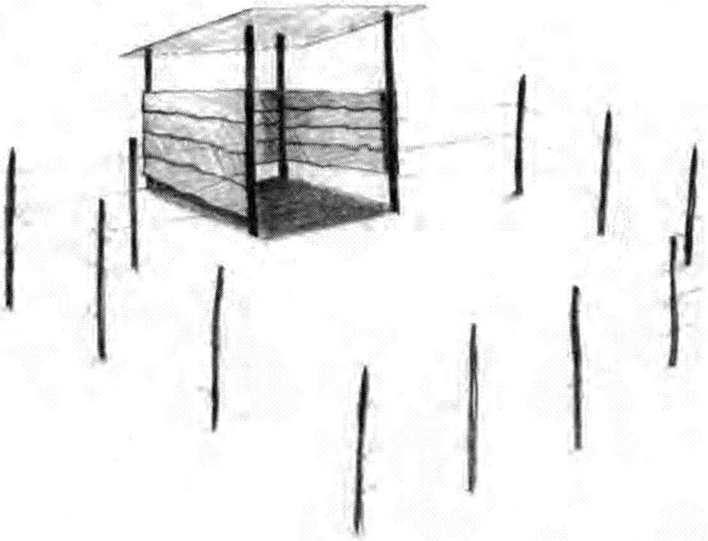

This building, called a "calf hutch" provides shade to animals in warm areas, while allowing good air flow. When it is cold, it can protect the animals from wind. The hutch should be a little less than 2 meters tall with a sloped roof.

If animals are exposed to bright sunlight or kept in poorly ventilated buildings for a long period of time, they may become overheated. This can cause many health problems including reproductive difficulties, respiratory distress, and slow growth. Cold weather exposure can have the same serious results.

Young animals in particular cannot adjust well to these extremes. In intense heat or cold, they may suffer more than older animals. With these animals, it is a good idea to allow the mother to protect her baby. In general, her instincts will be very reliable. But, it is also important to provide these animals with manmade shelter against extreme weather conditions.

Step 9. Separating Healthy and Sick Animals

Too often, diseases spread quickly from one animal to others on the same farm. Fortunately, if healthy animals are promptly removed from the pen of a sick animal, disease spread can often be prevented or slowed.

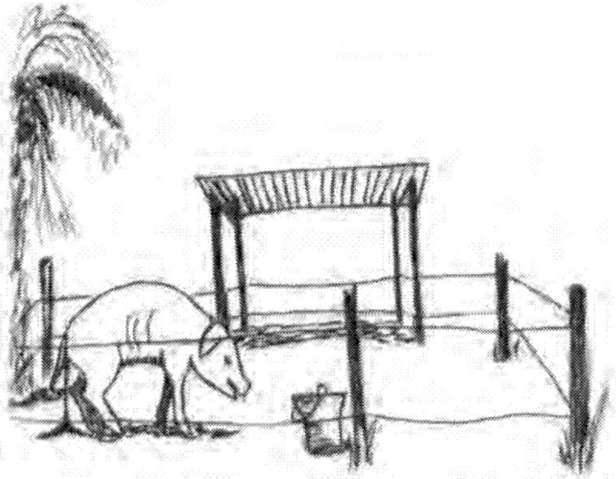

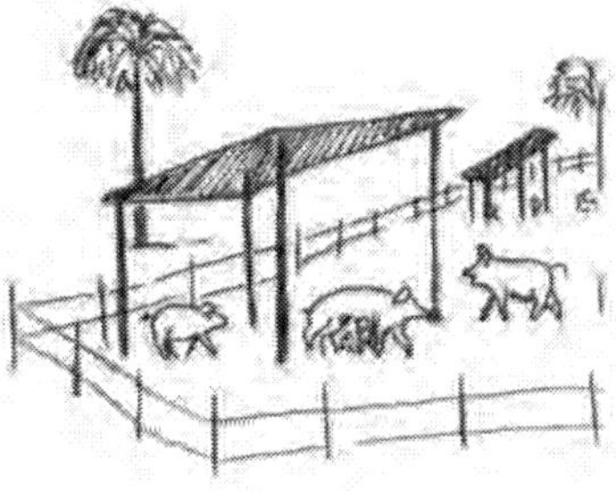

For example, many animals will develop diarrhea as babies. This condition, which can cause serious health problems, spreads quickly through a herd kept in the same pen. However, if the unaffected animals are separated from the animal with diarrhea, they are less likely to become ill.

Even though it may seem simpler to remove the sick animal from the pen, it is important to move the healthy animals to a fresh pen. Disease germs will stay in the pen where the sick animal was. They will still be able to infect healthy animals even if the sick animal is removed. So, to stop the spread, uninfected livestock should move to an area free of harmful germs.

This area should be far away from the sick animals' pen, at least 25 meters. If possible, move them even further since the disease may be able to spread through water, air, or feces.

Also, germs can remain on a sick animal's food and water troughs as well as on buildings in the affected pen. These items should not be moved to the clean pen. But, if they must be reused, they should be thoroughly cleaned and, if possible, disinfected.

After sickness is discovered in a group, their pen or pasture should not be used for six months or longer. This, along with the other precautions, will result in improved health for the entire farm.

Step10. Properly Disposing of Dead Animals

In addition to separating sick animals from the healthy livestock, properly disposing of dead animals will prevent the spread of disease.

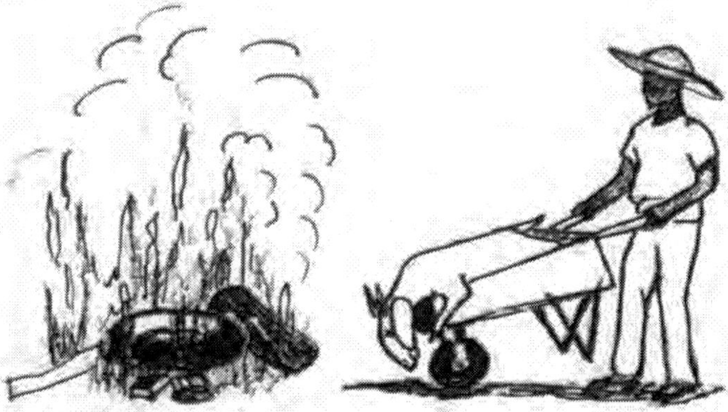

This farmer decides to burn the body of an animal that died from disease.

The bodies of animals that have died from illness can spread that sickness to others. Because of this, dead animals should be buried or burned quickly. This should be done at a safe distance from other animals.

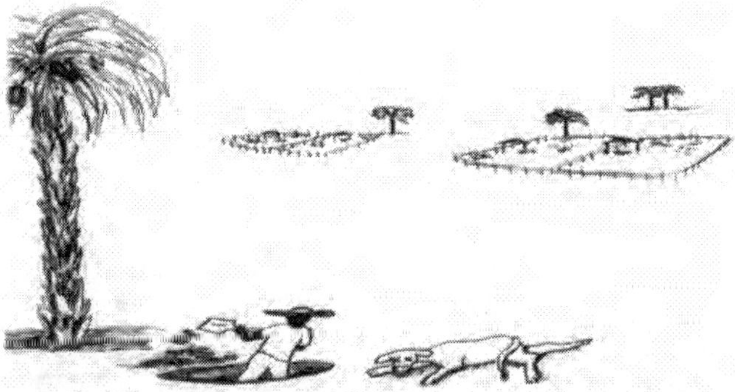

This farmer buries the dead body a safe distance from his livestock.

Not only will properly disposing of the bodies improve livestock health, it can also help reduce the spread of animal diseases to humans.

Section III

Special Notes on Poultry

Almost all of the principles that have been discussed so far can apply to poultry. Like all animals, they can have diseases or parasites. And, like all animals, there are ways to prevent many of these health problems.

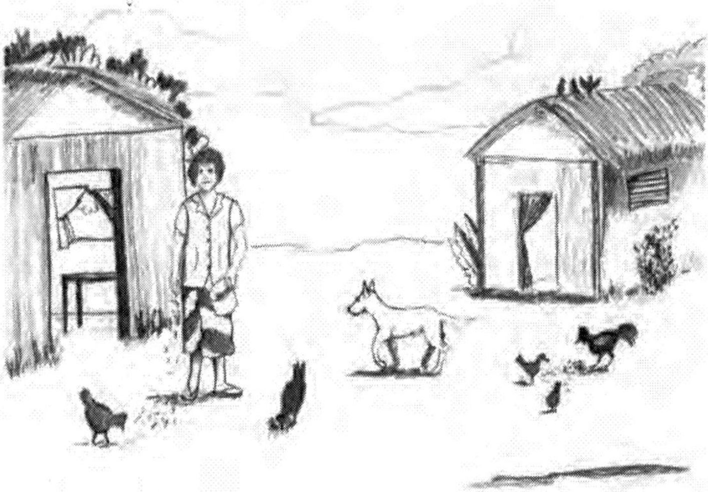

These chickens are being raised on the ground and ingest many dangerous germs. They are also likely to suffer from parasites.

Young poultry are especially susceptible to disease and parasites. So, in order to raise healthy poultry, special consideration must be given to the young. If they are kept on raised floor, they will be safe from many disease causing germs and parasites. There are many ways to build a raised floor. For instance, split bamboo, wood, and wire mesh are often used.

When an animal lives in a pen, separated from the soil, they no longer take in important vitamins and minerals from the soil. Also, the very small rocks (grit-gravel) that free ranging animals ingest are needed for good digestion. So, when birds are raised in pens, it is important to provide these animals proper nutrition. Poultry should be fed a finely ground, balanced diet with grit-gravel.

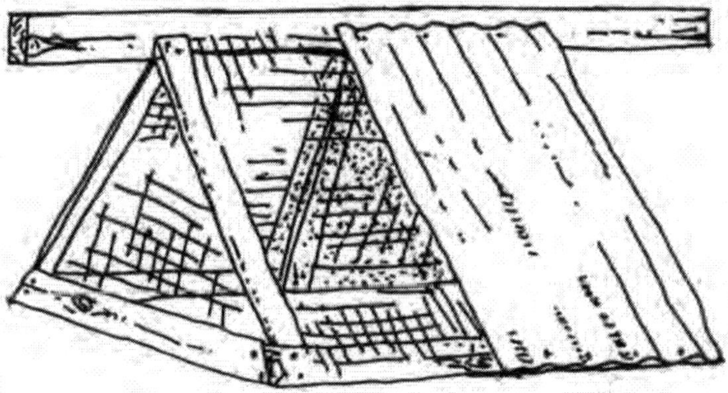

This building is called a "chicken tiller". It can be placed in one place for a few weeks and used to house chickens. The chickens will scratch the soil with their feet and their feces will fertilize the ground. After the tiller and the chickens are moved to a clean area, the fertilized land can be used to grow crops.

If it is impossible to keep young poultry on raised floors, they should live in areas where poultry haven't been raised before. If no space is available, house them in a place where poultry haven't lived recently. Remember, if temporary buildings and pens are used, animals will have fewer disease and parasite problems.

Too often, the same buildings or sheds are used for a very long time on some farms. Because of this, there will be many germs and parasite eggs in the soil. In these cases, it is almost impossible to raise healthy birds.

But, simply moving the poultry to new, clean building will greatly improve their health. And, if vaccines and parasite treatments are used, the birds will be even healthier.

Section IV

A Discussion on Raising Animals Off Ground

Raising animals in pens or buildings that are raised off the ground has many benefits. However, it is often impractical for a small farmer. The farmer must carefully decide if raised pens and buildings are right for his animals. Below are some issues to take into consideration when making this decision.

4.1 Drawbacks to Off Ground Animal Raising

The farmer and his assistants must understand how to build, maintain, and repair the pens and buildings. They must also be familiar with the special needs of animals that live in these pens and buildings.

Often, farmers are much more familiar with raising animals in regular pens and buildings, on the ground. So, these farmers can easily make small changes to improve their animals' health. It may be very difficult for these same farmers to make the switch to raised pens and buildings.

It can be expensive to buy the materials for building raised pens and structures, feeders, and waterers.

Animals that live in confined spaces need to be watched closely. Because they can't move freely, they must be moved out of the sun or away from cold winds.

The farmer must also provide these animals with nutrients and minerals. If they were free, they would find these nutrients in the soil. In confinement, on the other hand, their food intake is limited to whatever the farmer provides.

In confinement, animals cannot move away from feces or dirty areas. Sheds can be designed with floors that allow feces to drop through to the ground. Even then, feces must be removed frequently.

There are many other difficulties for specific animals. Baby pigs, for example, need iron to help with blood production. Usually, they can absorb it from the soil, especially in heavy reddish-yellow clay. If they are confined pens raised up, off the ground, they must receive expensive injections or the farmer must provide the iron rich clay immediately after birth. This is just one of many considerations for animals grown in pens that are raised up, off the ground.

4.2 Situations in Which Raising Animals Off Ground is Beneficial

On farms where most of the land is low and wet, a building that is raised up, off the ground, may be the only way to protect animals from disease causing germs and parasites.

Likewise, if most of a farmer's land has been used for a long time, it may be very dirty and contaminated with feces. Or, there may not be enough land to rotate pastures. In these cases, animals will benefit from off raised pens.

Even if raised pens and buildings are needed, a farmer can still use a system of rotation. Animals can be kept on the ground for half of the year and then confined in the pens for the growing season. Or, young animals can be kept separate, away from the grown animals. When they are weaned, they can be moved to regular pastures with the adults.

Farrowing Houses

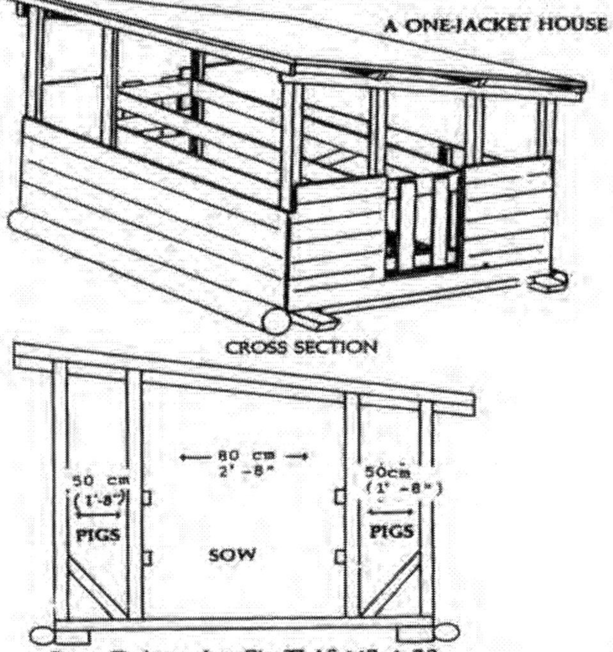

From: Tuskegee Ins. Cir. TI-AS-14B 6:79

This building is a good example of a raised building that keeps the livestock from contacting the ground or soil. It is built on runners for easy movement. Also, the floorboards are spaced so that feces and urine will fall to the ground. When the shed is moved, it will leave this dangerous filth behind.

Summary

There are simple and inexpensive steps that we can take to help our livestock be healthy and productive.

Step 1: *Ensure Good Location of Livestock & Poultry Facilities*
Try to use higher, well-drained areas for animals. In these areas a farmer may need to provide housing from extreme weather, along with provision of drinking water.

Step 2: *Manage Pens & Pastures Properly*
Periodically move animals and poultry from areas that have been in use for a long time. This allows time for disease germs and parasite eggs to die before they can infect animals.

Step 3: *Manage Pastures for Ruminants*
Alternating or "rotating" pastures gives the land time to recover and for the pasture to grow back. Also, when the land is left empty of livestock, particularly with exposure to sunlight, the immature parasites in the soil dry out and die.

Step 4: *Use Temporary & Movable Buildings*
If a farmer uses temporary or movable buildings, he can simply move the building to a fresh space where disease causing bacteria and parasites are not present.

Step 5: *Use the Cleanest Areas for Birthing*
Use of clean areas for birthing protects newborn animals from disease and parasites.

Step 6: *Provide Clean Drinking Water*
Dirty water is a common source of germs and parasites. Providing clean drinking protects livestock from this common source of infection.

Step 7: *Use Proper Feeding Techniques*
Food that is left on the ground often gets mixed with feces, germs and parasites. Using troughs, racks and other equipment keeps food off the ground and clean.

Step 8: *Protect Animals from Environmental Extremes*
Using well-ventilated buildings to protect livestock from extreme hot or cold is an important part of keeping them healthy.

Step 9: *Separate Healthy and Sick Animals*
Diseases can spread quickly from one animal to another. Sick animals should be separated from healthy animals to prevent diseases from spreading.

Step 10: *Properly Dispose of Dead Animals*
Dead animals should be buried or burned to prevent illness from spreading to other animals.

Christian Veterinary Mission (Publisher of this book)

Our vision is to see

Christ's love expressed through veterinary medicine.

Our mission is to

challenge, empower and facilitate veterinarians to serve through their profession, living out their Christian faith.

CVM also provides education and encouragement for those who desire to minister through service, prayer, relationship building, and modeling Christ's love.

About CVM

Christian Veterinary Mission (CVM) is a ministry registered non-profit Christian Service Organization 501(c)(3) based in Seattle, Washington, U.S.A.

CVM was founded in 1976 by Dr. Leroy Dorminy who came to realize the impact that veterinarians could have by integrating their faith with their practice, both locally and around the world. In 2008, CVM had nearly 30 veterinary professionals serving full-time internationally and over 200 veterinary professionals and student volunteers serve on short-term cross-cultural mission trips annually. CVM sponsors fellowship & prayer breakfasts at over 20 U.S. veterinary meetings each year and reaches out to veterinary students through Christian Veterinary Fellowship (CVF) groups in every veterinary school in the U.S. by encouraging them in spiritual growth and professional development.

There are over 3,500 veterinarians affiliated with CVM in the U.S. CVM also partners with organizations and networks in other countries that are focused on empowering Christian veterinarians. CVM has a volunteer advisory board of veterinarians who guide its vision, mission, and programming.

CVM books and the free International Animal Health Newsletter were written with small farmers, veterinarians, and agricultural development workers in mind. Our desire is that they would help individuals and groups develop an appropriate livestock program to meet community needs. CVM's Endowment Fund was started in the early years of the organization's life. The fund provides for meaningful programs that could not be funded by the regular budgeting process.

Made in the USA
Monee, IL
04 November 2026

67386136R00024